STRESS

calm

IN 7 MINUTES

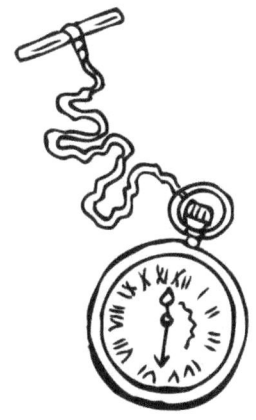

FOR NURSES

**BEVERLEY DENSHAM
& JANEY LEE GRACE**

McNIDDER & GRACE

Published by McNidder & Grace
21 Bridge Street
Carmarthen
SA31 3JS
Wales, UK

www.mcnidderandgrace.com

First published in 2024 © Beverley Densham and Janey Lee Grace

All rights reserved. No part of this work may be reproduced or transmitted in any form or by any means, electronic or mechanical, including photocopy, recording, or any information storage or retrieval system, without permission in writing from the publisher.

Beverley Densham and Janey Lee Grace have asserted their right to be identified as the authors of this work in accordance with the Copyright, Designs and Patents Act 1988.

The information given in this book is intended for general purposes only. It is not intended as and should not be relied upon as medical advice; always consult a medical practitioner. Any use of information in this book is at the reader's discretion and risk.

Every effort has been made to obtain necessary permission with reference to copyright material. The publisher apologises if, inadvertently, any sources remain unacknowledged and will be glad to make the necessary arrangements at the earliest opportunity.

A catalogue record for this work is available from the British Library.

ISBN 9780857162564 paperback
ISBN 9780857162571 ebook

Designer: JS Typesetting
Cover design: Tabitha Palmer

FOREWORD

Wow! This is such a great book for nurses who are looking for quick and effective strategies to alleviate stress. Time can fly during a shift and with the constant need to multitask and put the needs of our patients before our own we forget to look after ourselves. I currently work as a senior mental health practitioner, and I'm regularly exposed to traumatic stories, and situations. I know too well how difficult it can sometimes be to switch off after a shift.

I am currently leading on a wellbeing project for staff within my own service. My employer and the team always try to consider the wellbeing of ourselves as well as the wellbeing of our patients. There has certainly been a shift in views since I began my nursing career 18 years ago. We have 'wellbeing sessions' and we are encouraged to work with our patients outside, away from the clinical environment. I also like to share with my colleagues the recent benefits of becoming alcohol free – wine, it turns out wasn't the most effective coping strategy for me at the end of a busy shift!

The advice, strategies and exercises in this book are excellent and I'm certainly going to recommend these to my colleagues as well as continue to use the techniques during my working day.

A great read, perfect for busy nurses.

Andrew Blackman, 2024
Senior Mental Health Practitioner
Greater Manchester Mental Health NHS Foundation Trust

CONTENTS

Foreword		iii
Introduction: STRESS to Calm …		1
Chapter One	**Stress to Calm with Meditation**	15
	Tool 1. Let's Meditate	20
Chapter Two	**Stress to Calm with Positive Affirmations**	23
	Tool 2. Using Positive Affirmations	28
Chapter Three	**Stress to Calm with Neck and Shoulder Stretches**	31
	Tool 3. Stretching Your Neck and Shoulders	33
Chapter Four	**Stress to Calm with the Power Stretch**	37
	Tool 4. How to Power Stretch	40

Chapter Five	**Stress to Calm with Happiness**	43
	Tool 5. The Happy Exercise	47
Chapter Six	**Stress to Calm and the Power of Journaling**	51
	Tool 6. Grab a Pen and Journal	54
Chapter Seven	**Stress to Calm with Setting Goals and Visualisation**	57
	Tool 7. Reaching Your Goals Seeing the Success	60

Conclusion: CALM … 63

About the authors 69

References and further reading 71

INTRODUCTION
STRESS TO CALM …

If you've picked up this book, we're guessing it's because a part of you knows that your current stress levels are not sustainable. Something has to give!

Let us start by giving you hope that after reading this book, you will have some very simple tools that will help you to feel more in control and calmer. There are ways you can navigate the unique challenges you face in the nursing profession and while preserving your well-being.

When emotions start to run out of control, we will teach you to say – **just give me one minute!** And we will show you the one-minute tools that will make you feel so much better, and quickly.

For many of us, stress has become an inevitable part of our lives. From managing work deadlines to balancing personal commitments, we can easily become overwhelmed and consumed by stress. And for nurses, this stress can be compounded by the responsibility of a heavy workload and long hours, a lack of adequate staffing and funds, as well as the demanding nature of the work.

Stress is often viewed as a negative experience that should be avoided or minimised at all costs. But it's a common myth that stress is always bad for us. Stress is a natural response to challenging situations and can be helpful in certain circumstances. In fact, the release of cortisol, a stress hormone, is a necessary physiological reaction that allows us to react quickly in dangerous or stressful situations, such as the 'fight or flight' response. Where it goes wrong, is when we perceive our bulging file of work to take home as a predator about to attack!

When we encounter a stressful situation, our body releases cortisol, adrenaline and other hormones that trigger a series of physical responses. These responses include an increase in heart rate, blood pressure and breathing rate, which prepares the body to respond quickly to the threat. This physiological response is useful when there is a real physical threat, such as being chased by a tiger. Our ancestors needed that ability to focus on their escape … and fast! Sadly, we have the same response in our modern world. But in the hospital, in the consulting

Introduction: Stress to Calm ...

room, surrounded by colleagues and patients, even when back home – there are no tigers!

The heart can be pounding, the 'threat' feels very real, but this full stress response is inappropriate. What we are confronting may genuinely be a big problem – concerns about patient care or needing to stay on duty after your shift has finished – and there may seemingly be no positive solutions, but it isn't life-threatening to you, it isn't a real and present danger for you, and so these physical responses can have negative consequences on our well-being. We aren't meant to constantly release these chemicals, and the prolonged exposure to cortisol and other stress hormones can lead to physical and emotional health problems over time, including anxiety, depression, high blood pressure and a weakened immune system. It can lead to burnout and fatigue, making it difficult to function effectively in our daily lives. In addition to the physical impact, when our minds are consumed with panic, destructive thoughts and incessant chatter, we can fall into patterns of negative thinking which can impact our mental health and overall outlook on life.

We want you to feel empowered and in control in your professional capacity – and these simple tools we share with you in this book will help you find more of a sense of calm. They will help you manage the stresses in your working day, help you find your centre and maintain balance in your working day. These tools are practical and based on scientifically proven methods that will reduce stress, empower you to take control of your stress levels and improve your overall wellbeing.

The tools in this book are designed to be easily incorporated into a busy nurse's daily routine. They can be done in just a few minutes a day and they require no special equipment or training. We will explore techniques such as breathing exercises, mindfulness, positive affirmations and visualisation, all of which have been shown to reduce stress and promote calm.

We will explore the concept of choosing happiness. Yes, we show you that this can be a choice! We look at the importance of setting goals for both work and personal life. We also learn to focus on positive outcomes and how to take small steps towards achieving them, to shift your mindset and cultivating a more positive outlook.

Throughout the book, we will cite scientific studies that demonstrate the benefits of each technique we discuss. For example, studies have shown that mindfulness can reduce stress and anxiety levels, while breathing exercises can lower cortisol levels and improve heart health.

Introduction: Stress to Calm ...

We hope you will be able to utilise the real and tangible benefits of these simple tools and techniques.

Nursing is undoubtedly one of the most demanding (albeit rewarding) professions, requiring not only technical skills but also emotional resilience. The healthcare landscape is constantly evolving, and nurses are at the forefront of patient care, often working long hours in high-pressure environments, so it comes as no surprise that nursing is consistently ranked among the most stressful professions.

A report 'Staff Stress and Wellbeing in the NHS' (2018) by the Health and Safety Executive specifically explored stress and well-being in the NHS, including nursing staff. The findings indicated that high levels of demand, coupled with low levels of control and support, contributed to stress among NHS employees, including nurses.

Among these, heavy workloads, inadequate staffing, and the emotional toll of dealing with patients' suffering were contributors to nurses' stress levels. In addition, the unpredictable nature of healthcare, coupled with the responsibility of making critical decisions in real-time, adds another layer of stress.

Florence Nightingale, once said, *'The very first requirement in a hospital is that it should do the sick no harm.'* This underlines the immense responsibility that nurses bear for the well-being of their patients. Nursing professor and author, Jean Watson, emphasizes the transformative power of compassion in nursing. She notes, *'Caring for others is an expression of what it means to be fully human.'* We acknowledge that there is a noble aspect to nursing, but this also highlights the emotional weight that comes with the profession.

So why *are* nurse's feeling the need to go from Stress to Calm?

As already alluded to, heavy workloads, often with insufficient staffing levels, whether due to budget constraints or shortages of qualified personnel, contribute significantly to stress and several nurses felt that it can lead to burnout, and compromised patient care. Nurses face emotional demands: dealing with patients who are in pain, experiencing trauma, or facing life-threatening conditions can take a toll on nurses emotionally. Nurses are expected to have a huge amount of compassion, but the constant exposure to suffering and trauma can lead to emotional exhaustion.

Some nurses felt that within the NHS there is a lack of, or limited access to essential resources, such as medical equipment, medications, or proper training, and several

Introduction: Stress to Calm ...

cited the burden of administrative tasks that take time away from patient care. It seems that excessive paperwork, charting requirements, and bureaucratic processes can contribute to stress and frustration. Ineffective communication, both within the healthcare team and with patients, also creates misunderstandings and contributes to workplace stress.

Nurses also told us that in recent years they face ethical dilemmas that create moral distress. Balancing patient autonomy, family expectations, and institutional policies can be challenging, leading to internal conflict and stress. It is of course, the nature of the job, but shift work and irregular schedules, night shifts, etc. causes disruption to circadian rhythms and the challenge of balancing work and personal life can contribute to stress.

We were surprised to find that nurses, despite their crucial role in patient care, may sometimes feel undervalued and unappreciated. Lack of acknowledgment for their hard work can contribute to feelings of stress and burnout.

Former nurse, and author Ann Girling, documents her stress and burnout as a nurse, her depression, baby loss and grief journey, in her book *Journey to Chocolate*. Ann talks of exhaustion, anger, having a short fuse, smoking, drinking alcohol, and overwhelm at work. Ann says:

'I worked in the NHS as a nurse and then as a health visitor for 30 years, that was 20 years ago and I suspect it's got worse rather than better: due to the size of caseloads, micromanagement from managers without our clinical knowledge, constant change, no money and concerns about quality of care and our fear of missing something critical, e.g. child abuse. I definitely brought stress home ... all the above was poor!'

What are the main problems nurses face – and why is this profession prone to stress? We asked some nurses in an independent survey and their responses were all very much the same. They told us about being short staffed and feeling they are not getting everything done to a high enough standard, suffering from chronic insomnia and being prone to overthinking. We have changed all names to protect their identity.

Regina was a Registered Nurse, Sister in an Emergency Department and has recently retired. She said that they were always short staffed, there was a lack of equipment and not enough facilities to cater for increasing numbers of patients. Regina said she felt unable to switch off from work which affected her sleep and general lifestyle, and if her **employer** did offer any help, it was difficult to access when working shifts with short breaks.

Introduction: Stress to Calm ...

Felicity has been a Registered Nurse for 32 years. She told us there was immense pressure to get everything done in too short a time. She says despite having a good diet and exercise, the stresses caused by the job means she drinks too much, resulting in poor sleep, often waking at 4 am.

Sadie is a Registered Nurse who is a Care Home Manager and has been in management for 10 years, nursing for 29 years.

'As a manager I have additional stress about staffing levels, budgets, bed occupancy, compliance with regulators, etc. There are peaks and troughs, some quiet weeks, and weeks when you have staff off sick, no cover available and you're still trying to meet the usual daily demands.'

It's tough, even for those in management roles.

Dominic has been a Registered General Nurse for three years. He says, *'I'm stressed because I'm not able to be the nurse I want to be due to time constraints and workload. I work in a private sector hospital, so the pressures aren't quite the same as the NHS, but still similar issues arise. I would never go back to the NHS though!'*

And the issues arise in the private sector too, and not just within the NHS!

Nikki has been a Practice Nurse and Respiratory Specialist for 28 years.

She describes a workload that is heavy and pressured. Constant requests from reception and GP to fit in extra patients when time is already fully allocated. Nikki says: *'We become subject to patients anger and frustration over difficulties with accessing all NHS patient services. I find I'm regularly not getting breaks, finishing late and I'm constantly expected to work outside of my role without adequate time being allocated.'*

It's tough for specialists too.

Nikki admits that she brings her stress home, she says she can't switch off straight away, often she feels the need to vent, let off steam or have a good cry.

Reading some parts of this survey made us want to cry! But we can do some small things to find calm amidst the chaos. Recognizing the undeniable stress faced by nursing, it becomes so important to equip nurses with effective coping strategies.

A study published in the *Journal of Nursing Management* found that nurses with a supportive workplace culture that encourages open communication and teamwork has been proven to alleviate stress among nursing staff.

Workplace support seemed patchy in our survey, and one nurse said:

'There is an external HR company recommended to us who offer a counselling service, but I don't know anyone who has tried to access this. You are also recommended to talk with your team leaders or senior GP's, but time is always pressured so it's difficult to access their time. There are team meetings where some things can be discussed as a form of group support, but this usually takes place on zoom with no opportunity for private discussion. After a major incident those involved do get to discuss in private soon after the incident, but we usually only get a short time before either we go back to work or go home… and that's it!

It would help if there was someone available for face-to-face support and could be accessed a few days a week. Someone to talk through your issues with and who could help you to talk to your employer if needed. Or just individual time allocated even once a month for individuals/ groups to be face to face purely for emotional support and to check in on our well-being.'

If you are a manager – please take note!

So, it's a mixed bag regarding workplace support for nurses but what we hope is that we can show you some simple tools that can be incorporated into your daily life, at home and at work, and will make a real difference.

The tools – the lowdown

We will cover some techniques in this book that you will already be aware of, and some that might be new to you. Everyone has heard of meditation (though you may not realise how to do it or that even one minute of meditation can be beneficial). You may be aware that stretching, good posture and breathing techniques can help with stress. You may have come across the Power Pose, which we can't wait to share with you, and you may be aware of the power of positive affirmations, or journaling. In any case, we will give you the lowdown on why these practices can work so well to relieve stress, and we give you very simple versions that can be done anywhere and in one minute or less!

A word about *mindfulness*, which is not one of the designated practices in this book. You may wonder why. It's become rather a catch-all term in recent years, but we would hope that you can practise mindfulness almost without trying, when you use these tools.

Mindfulness is the practice of intentionally focusing your attention on the present moment. It involves paying attention to your thoughts, feelings and bodily sensations, in a non-judgmental way. Mindfulness has been shown to be an effective way to reduce stress and anxiety and it can help you to improve your focus and concentration. We think that all the tools and techniques we share in this book could come under the banner of 'being mindful'.

How to use this book

Each short chapter gives you a stress to calm technique that should take only one minute per day. Put these seven one-minute techniques together from each of the seven chapters and you will have a set of tools that takes just seven minutes!

In an ideal world you could read each of the short chapters and then start using them straight away – ideally all seven every day – but you can of course pick out any that appeal and just give it a go, whenever suits you.

In time you can adapt these techniques and use the ones that work for you best. We appreciate that you may not want to be punching the air in the hospital ward or adopting a power pose as you stand in front of a patient(!), but you can always find a moment to fit these tools into your day.

But if you are someone who likes to flick through, or even start at the back of the book – **we see you** – that's fine too.

It's as easy as saying: **Just give me one minute!** and then using that minute to try any one of these tools and then notice if repetition begins to make a difference.

We would love to know how you get on, so do send any feedback to us. You'll find our contact details are towards the end of this book.

CHAPTER ONE

STRESS TO CALM WITH MEDITATION

Tip: Remember it's just ONE minute – you do NOT have to levitate!

What's the lowdown?

All of us have heard of meditation, and many of us have tried it – but given up when we realised that sitting for 20 minutes while our mind wandered off to write shopping lists or worry about our next work project, might not suit us. The reality is when you find a way to meditate that works, it's liberating, and as we are going to show here, it can take as little as one minute.

Meditation is a powerful tool that can help to reduce stress, improve mental clarity and bring a sense of calm and balance to our lives. Contrary to popular belief, meditation does not have to be done in a certain way or for a certain length of time. Even a minute or so of meditation per day can be hugely beneficial for calming the mind and reducing stress.

One of the primary benefits of meditation is its ability to help us manage stress. When we are stressed, our bodies release a hormone called cortisol, which can have negative effects on our health if it is consistently elevated. However, studies have shown that regular meditation can help to reduce cortisol levels, which in turn can lead to a reduction in stress and anxiety.

Meditation can also help to improve mental clarity and focus. It helps us with mindfulness and being more present, more in the moment. We become more aware of our thoughts and emotions and learn to better manage them. This can lead to a greater sense of inner peace and clarity and can help us to approach our daily tasks with greater focus and more productivity.

> **'Through meditation and by giving full attention to one thing at a time, we can learn to direct attention where we choose.'**
> Eknath Easwaran, spiritual teacher

There are many ways to meditate, and it is important to find a method that works for you. Some people prefer to sit on a mat or a cushion, while others prefer to lie down or sit in a chair. The key is to find a comfortable position that allows you to relax and focus your mind. You absolutely can utilise your time on the train or bus!

Let go of the idea that it must be a long session sitting cross-legged.

One popular method of meditation is mindfulness meditation, which involves focusing on the present moment and observing your thoughts and emotions without judgment.

To practise *mindfulness meditation*, find a quiet place to sit or lie down and focus on your breath. Notice the sensations of your breath as it enters and exits your body and allow your thoughts to come and go without getting caught up in them. It's that simple!

Another method of meditation is *guided meditation*, which involves listening to a recorded meditation that guides you through the process. This can be especially helpful for beginners because it provides structure and support as you learn to quiet your mind and focus your attention.

Meditation can be incorporated into your daily routine, even if you are busy or at work. For example, you can take a few minutes to focus on your breath and observe your thoughts and emotions during a break. You can also try a *walking meditation*, which involves focusing on the sensations of your body as you walk and being fully present in the moment.

You will obviously have your eyes open as you walk, but meditation can be done with eyes open. This is called (not surprisingly) *open-eye meditation* or *focused attention meditation* and is a technique that involves maintaining a relaxed and focused state of mind while keeping your eyes open and fixating your gaze on an object or a point. This can be a helpful practice for those who want to integrate mindfulness into their daily routine.

You could try simply focusing on your breath wherever you are. Take a few deep breaths and then focus your attention on your breath and then continue to work. Whenever your mind starts to wander or you feel distracted, bring your attention back to your breath. This can help you reduce stress and increase productivity by bringing more focus and clarity to your work. The key is to maintain a relaxed and focused state of mind while keeping your eyes open and fixating your gaze on an object or your breath. With practice, open-eye meditation can be just as effective as traditional meditation for reducing stress and promoting overall wellbeing.

Many people have spoken about the benefits of meditation. Oprah Winfrey described meditation as a transformative practice that has helped her to manage stress and stay grounded.

Many scientific studies have demonstrated the benefits of meditation. One study published in the journal *Frontiers in Human Neuroscience* found that just four days of mindfulness meditation led to significant improvements in mood and working memory capacity. Another study, published in the *Journal of Alternative and Complementary Medicine*, found that mindfulness meditation led to significant reductions in anxiety and depression.

So, don't knock this one till you have tried it!

Meditation really is a powerful tool that can help to reduce stress, improve mental clarity and bring a sense of calm and balance to our lives. If you find your mind wandering off the first few times you try it, just relax, it's OK! Let go of the idea that we must clear our mind of all thoughts; that's unlikely to happen. What is possible, though, is that we show up anyway, consciously focus on our breath and observe the thoughts that pop up, and then we can reap the many benefits that meditation has to offer.

A word about breathing

We all breathe … of course we do, but it's enlightening when we realise that just by becoming conscious of the way we are breathing, we can almost instantly reduce our anxiety. Our breath is a reaction to our mental state:

when we are stressed, we breathe too fast, and can even hyperventilate.

We can proactively slow down our breathing. Controlling our breath will have a direct effect on us at a psychological level: it can help with hormone function, reduce inflammation, release endorphins and calm anxiety.

Simply by focusing on our breath and practising different breath work exercises, we can regulate our nervous system, slow down our heart rate, and improve our overall sense of wellbeing, we may become happier because of the naturally released neurotransmitters.

Leading breath work practitioner Tim Van de Vliet says: 'If you can control your breath, you control your life.'

By focusing on our breath and practising different techniques, we can regulate our nervous system and improve our ability to cope with stress.

TOOL 1

Let's Meditate – give me just one minute!

You can enjoy this at your desk, sitting, standing, or lying down. You can even sneak off to the staffroom or toilet (if that's the only private space you can find) for a quiet minute to do this!

Before you start, check in with how you are feeling in relation to your stress levels.

You may want to select a level from 0 (feeling completely fine) to 10 (feeling very stressed). What level are you at this moment?

If you are sitting, please don't sit like a banana – i.e. bent over! Sit with good posture, with your bottom at the back of the chair, with your feet hip-width apart, and with your head, neck, shoulders and back relaxed.

If you're standing, stand with good posture – with a natural curve of your spine, with your feet hip-width apart and a slight bend in your knees. Look forwards and relax your arms down by your side.

Lie down if you have the luxury of a private space and it's comfortable for you, and if you want more back support, bend your knees, again with your feet hip-width apart.

Close your eyes, focus and concentrate on your breathing. Take 10 relaxing breaths in and out – in through your nose and out through your mouth – and relax with each breath. Feel your tummy rise and fall. Relax as you breathe in and out. Relax your head, neck and shoulders, then relax your back, hips and thighs, relax your legs, feet and toes, relax your arms, hands and fingers. By the end of the 10 breaths your whole body should feel relaxed.

Say 'Well done' to yourself during the breathing exercise, out loud or silently; both work well as an affirmation.

You can set an alarm for 1 minute for this meditation exercise or simply enjoy 10 relaxing breaths in and out.

Think about how you feel afterwards.

Check in to see if the stress level number you selected before you did the exercise has reduced.

CHAPTER TWO

STRESS TO CALM WITH POSITIVE AFFIRMATIONS

Tip: Remember it's just ONE minute – and you can have a CALM day!

What's the lowdown?

Positive affirmations are statements or phrases that are repeated with the intention of instilling a positive belief or attitude. The idea behind positive affirmations is that by repeating these positive statements, we can change our subconscious thought patterns, and ultimately our behaviour and emotions. Positive affirmations can work to reduce stress by helping to reframe negative thought patterns and shift our focus to positive beliefs and outcomes.

Our unconscious mind is not wired to focus on the positive, which is why many people find it difficult to introduce positive affirmations into their daily routine. The human brain tends to be wired to focus on threats and negative stimuli as a survival mechanism – we are on the lookout for danger! However, with consistent practice, positive affirmations can help to rewire the brain and promote positive thinking and emotional regulation.

Author Louise Hay wrote extensively on the power of positive affirmations. She believed that affirmations could help individuals to release negative thought patterns and improve mental and physical wellbeing. There are several scientific studies that support the effectiveness of positive affirmations for reducing stress and promoting wellbeing.

Some simple ways to introduce positive affirmations into your daily routine include writing them down, repeating them out loud, picking out a positive affirmation card, or visualising them during meditation or relaxation exercises.

'You are imperfect, you are wired for struggle, but you are worthy of love and belonging.'
Brené Brown, writer

You have probably heard of the idea of repeating positive affirmations/statements about yourself, to make you feel more positive. Sadly our unconscious mind has a strong bullshit detector! If we state something that feels too far-fetched for us – 'I am incredibly beautiful!' – our inner critic may tell us, 'No you're not.' So, if you tell yourself 'I am relaxed' when you are chilling at home, you may believe the affirmation, but if you're at work and feeling stressed and anxious, this affirmation probably won't work, we can't lie to ourselves! Unless, that is, you first take some action to make it feel possible. For example, you could use the meditation tool in Chapter One, which can help you change your state quickly from a stressed to a calmer state, with the result that the 'I am relaxed' affirmation will feel relevant and effective.

It might feel like too much of a stretch to declare: 'I am enthusiastic and full of energy', but you could consider what that affirmation means to you, and why it feels important.

Later in this book (see page 51), we talk about journaling, and how writing down what affirmations means to you can help. Let's take a quick peek now. For example, if you aren't feeling full of energy, you could jot down in your notebook: 'How can I find more energy? What action steps am I going to take to improve my energy levels?' We will teach you how to respond/react to these questions. Sometimes it might be as simple as getting a good night's sleep, getting to bed earlier and relaxing before you go to sleep.

We must consciously choose to repeat positive affirmations. Sadly, the negative statements often flow in our thoughts more easily, but we should be conscious of that too. When we repeatedly say: 'I am stressed,' we are instructing our unconscious mind to keep us in that state of stress.

It helps to start noticing your negative thoughts and ask if there is something that could turn them around. Perhaps you just need a two-minute break to breathe and do some stretching or take a walk and get some fresh air. Or maybe you need some form of connection with others, to talk to one of your work colleagues or to seek help from a professional about what is on your mind.

Positive Affirmation cards can help. These are a set of cards with statements that help prompt you to think about something positive. If you have a set of Positive Affirmation cards, pick one out and consider what the message means to you. If you are picking a positive affirmation with a friend, family or work colleague, talk to each other about what this positive affirmation means to you, then swap over. It can lead into interesting conversations, enabling you to laugh or talk about things you need to get off your chest.

Positive affirmations help you to challenge yourself to

think, speak, write and behave more positively at work and at home.

An affirmation can also be used like a mantra, to be repeated to give you more confidence in a situation outside of your comfort zone, such as needing to speak up to your management. You might say to yourself: 'I can do this' or 'It's going to be OK.' Choose a positive statement that feels good to you.

'The greater the obstacle, the more glory in overcoming it.'

Molière (Jean-Baptiste Poquelin), actor and playwright

There are several scientific studies that support the effectiveness of positive affirmations for reducing stress and promoting wellbeing. For example, a study by Moser *et al.* (2016) found that participants who practised self-affirmation exercises reported lower levels of stress and greater emotional resilience in response to a stressful task. Another study by Latham and Locke (2007) found that individuals who used positive self-talk and affirmations were more likely to achieve their goals and experience greater levels of success and wellbeing.

Practise this. Practice makes … not exactly perfect, but it will lead to an improvement in your stress levels.

Repeating the practice of using positive affirmation or using positive affirmation cards on a daily or regular basis really can make a real difference.

A study published by the US National Library of Medicine suggests that incorporating self-affirmations into a daily routine can be a powerful tool for improving mental and emotional wellbeing, reducing stress and promoting personal growth. According to the study, affirmations can reduce stress, improve wellbeing, enhance academic performance and make people more open to behaviour change. The study also recommends using positive, truthful statements as affirmations, such as 'I get on well with my child/children, mum and sister.' This kind of affirmation can be especially helpful when dealing with challenging or negative situations involving specific people or relationships.

TOOL 2

Using Positive Affirmations – give me just one minute!

Using positive affirmations can be done at work or home, with a work colleague, friend or family or on your own.

Pick an affirmation from the list below:

I am calm, I am loved, I am surrounded by love.

I learn from my mistakes. I learn from mine and other people's mistakes.

I think positive words. When negativity appears, I find a solution, talk to those I trust and choose positivity.

It's going to be OK.

I can have fun, I am happy.

I am creative.

I enjoy exercise.

I always have lots of good ideas.

I am energetic.

I radiate positive energy wherever I go.

I am healthy.

I have good relationships.

I am strong.

I am kind.

I am grateful.

I am myself, it's OK to be myself.

I enjoy spending time with friends or family and have good relationships.

I am peaceful.

Repeat the positive affirmation you have chosen to yourself 3 times.

Think about what this means to you today.

If you don't feel what the affirmation is describing, ask yourself, *How can I feel more like this affirmation today? Are there any action steps for me to take to feel more like this affirmation to improve my life or work?*

Write down what tips and action steps you came up with.

Don't feel impatient or irritated with yourself if you don't feel like you should when repeating the affirmation. Think about how you can put steps in place in your life and work to make this feeling happen.

You can do this exercise with someone else by picking an affirmation from the list and then each of you have a turn talking about what the positive affirmation message means to you.

CHAPTER THREE

STRESS TO CALM WITH NECK AND SHOULDER STRETCHES

Tip: Remember it's just ONE minute – and you will feel GREAT after a big stretch!

What's the lowdown?

Stretching is a simple yet effective way to reduce stress, improve flexibility and alleviate back pain. It's good for emotional wellbeing too. Most of us know this or do this automatically – like doing a big stretch and a yawn when we first wake up. You will notice dogs do this intuitively and are good at stretching. In yoga there is a pose called Downward Dog! Young children naturally stretch a lot too, instinctively knowing that it's good for their body, but sadly we tend to forget as we get older or get out of the habit of doing it, especially if we are working. Instead of stretching, and sitting with good posture, we tend to tighten everything up, and then wonder why we feel like a coiled spring!

When we sit for extended periods, our muscles tend to tighten, causing discomfort and stiffness. When we are bending down or lifting this can cause strain on our muscles too. Stretching helps to loosen these muscles, improving blood flow and oxygenation, which can help to reduce stress and anxiety. Stretching can help to improve posture too, which can reduce the likelihood of developing back pain.

In terms of physical benefits, stretching has been shown to increase flexibility, improve range of motion and reduce the risk of injury. A study published in *The Journal of Strength and Conditioning Research* found that stretching for just 30 seconds improved flexibility and range of motion in participants. Additionally, a study published in the *Clinical Journal of Sports Medicine* found that stretching reduced the risk of injury in athletes.

> **'Life is like riding a bicycle. To keep your balance, you must keep moving.'**
> Albert Einstein

Stretching can also have emotional benefits. A study published in the *International Journal of Workplace Health Management* found that stretching at work can improve mood, reduce stress and increase job satisfaction. Another study published in the *Journal of Bodywork and*

Movement Therapies found that stretching can help to reduce anxiety and depression.

Stretching well does not require a gym session and simple stretches that can be done in any small space can be beneficial. Neck stretches, shoulder stretches, and wrist stretches can all be done anywhere but you may prefer to sneak into a private space, the staffroom, supply cupboard, etc. Stretching can be done whenever you have some spare time – how about stretching while waiting for your bus! Even a minute of stretching can have benefits, and it can be done anywhere, making it an accessible and convenient self-care practice.

It's worth mentioning that being conscious of your breathing as you stretch helps too.

TOOL 3

Stretching Your Neck and Shoulders – give me just one minute!

To begin with, let's just keep it simple. Start by breathing in and out slowly and begin to follow the instructions below.

Shoulder circles

Sit or stand with good posture and with your eyes looking forward. Set an alarm for 1 minute.

Relax your arms down by your side, and circle both your shoulders 5 times backwards, lifting the shoulders up and back and round in a circular small movement. Then circle both your shoulders 5 times forward, again in small circular movements.

This will loosen your shoulders and upper body and make you feel more relaxed.

Neck stretches

• Tilt

Relax your arms down by your side. Tilt your head to the side (as if moving your ear down towards your shoulder) and feel the stretch in the side of the neck, and then tilt the head to the other side. Listen to your body, moving only as far as is comfortable for you; it's a small, slow, controlled movement. Repeat 3 times each side.

Breathe naturally, breathing in through your nose and moving on the out breath. As you exhale move and hold, then breathe in and go back to the starting position.

- **Chin to chest**

Relax your arms down by your side. Sitting or standing with good posture, slowly bring your chin towards your chest to gently stretch your neck to mid back muscles, then bring your head back to the starting position.

Breathe naturally, breathing in through your nose and moving on the out breath. As you exhale, move and hold, then breathe in and go back to the starting position.

- **Turn**

Relax your arms down by your side. Sitting or standing with good posture, slowly turn your head one way, and then turn your head the other way. Repeat this 2–5 times.

Breathe naturally, breathing in through your nose and moving on the out breath. As you exhale, move and hold, then breathe in and go back to the starting position.

Notice how much better you feel after these simple stretches.

Bonus Tools

As you do your stretches, you can either breathe naturally or, if you want to try something a little more complex, you can focus on a style of breathing that is taught in Pilates, called 'lateral thoracic breathing'. Put your hands on your rib cage and take a deep breath through the nose, feeling the breath inside and to the back of your body. You should feel your ribs pushing your hands outward as you breathe in.

If you want to develop your breathing technique, try deep breathing. This involves taking slow, deep breaths from the diaphragm, filling your lungs with air and then exhaling slowly. Breathe into the tummy and let your tummy rise and fall as you breathe. Research has found that deep breathing can lower your stress and anxiety levels and improve your feeling of wellbeing.

You could also try the 4-7-8 breathing technique. This involves inhaling for 4 seconds, holding your breath for 7 seconds and exhaling for 8 seconds. A study published by the *Journal of Alternative and Complementary Medicine* found this technique can help reduce stress and improve sleep quality.

Next time you can't sleep, give this a try and see if it works for you!

CHAPTER FOUR

STRESS TO CALM WITH THE POWER STRETCH

Tip: Remember it's just ONE minute – and you can FEEL the power!

What's the lowdown?

If we are feeling stressed, or a bit blue, our body tends to reflect that: everything seems to 'go downward.' We can find ourselves putting our head in our hands, slumping over and generally slipping down our chair, or hunching over if we are standing up.

It's possible to make a conscious choice to be happy, and literally change the way you feel, or change your state of mind.

We know there is a link between body and mind, and just a fearful thought can have a physiological effect on our body. Ever felt fearful and needed to run to the loo? Unconsciously our body reacts to stress in strange ways, impacting our thoughts and emotions, but we can consciously use our body to impact our thoughts and emotions in a positive way.

The mind-body connection that explores the relationship between our thoughts, emotions and physical sensations is well researched. We've heard it described as the Cybernetic Loop – the idea that the mind affects the body, but the body can affect the mind.

Let's explore this further. Have you heard of the Power Pose? It's about assuming a posture that conveys confidence, strength and assertiveness. By consciously adopting certain postures, we can positively impact our mental state and improve our sense of self-assurance.

'I am not afraid; I was born to do this.'
Joan of Arc

Research conducted by social psychologist Amy Cuddy, who gave a very popular TED Talk called 'Your body language may shape who you are', explored the effects of power poses on an individual's feelings of power, confidence and performance. Studies indicated that adopting high-power poses such as standing tall with an open posture and outstretched arms for a brief period can lead to increased feelings of power and reduced stress levels.

By adopting a power pose, we can alter hormone levels, increase testosterone (associated with dominance and confidence) and decrease cortisol (a stress hormone). These hormonal changes may contribute to the reported psychological effects.

The jury is out as to what extent we will increase testosterone just by standing up! But the broader concept of the mind-body connection is well-established. Our physical state can influence our mental state, and vice versa.

How does posture impact on our happiness?

The concept of choosing happiness involves recognising happiness as a choice that we can make in any moment, regardless of external circumstances. (More on this in Chapter Five.)

By changing our thoughts and focusing on positive emotions, we can move from feeling stressed to feeling calm in a very short space of time. Posture can also play a role in this process, as adopting a more upright and confident posture can help to improve mood and reduce stress.

Studies have shown that choosing happiness and changing our state can have a range of benefits. One study published in the journal *Emotion* found that adopting a more upright and open body posture can increase feelings of power and confidence, leading to more positive emotions.

By taking back control over our unconscious mind and changing our body posture to feel happier, we can improve our wellbeing and reduce stress in a short space of time. By focusing on positive emotions and engaging in activities that promote happiness, we can cultivate a more positive outlook and improve our overall quality of life.

TOOL 4

How to Power Stretch – give me just one minute!

You can do this sitting or standing.

If you are sitting, think of your posture, with your bottom at the back of the chair, feet hip-width apart, your head, neck and shoulders and back relaxed and looking forwards.

If you're standing, stand with good posture, with a natural curve of your spine, your feet hip-width apart and a slight bend in your knees, and looking forwards.

Stress to Calm with the Power Stretch

First, place your hands on your hips.

Then place your hands at the side of your neck; do not poke your head forwards. Gently squeeze your elbows back until you feel a gentle or good stretch in your chest and shoulders; this also strengthens your mid back muscles.

Raise your arms in the air above you, wherever is comfortable for you, and then bring your arms back down and place your hands back on your hips again.

You can breathe naturally, or you can add some breathing into the exercise by following the instruction below.

Breathe in through your nose. As you breathe out through your mouth, place your hands at the side of your neck and squeeze your elbows back until you feel a gentle stretch in your chest and shoulders.

As you move your arms up in the air, breathe in through the nose. As you exhale, float your arms back down, placing your hands back on your hips.

Repeat – 5 times or for one minute.

This exercise will help to improve posture and release muscles, stretching your chest and shoulders, strengthening mid back, and helping you to feel more confident, happier and more powerful.

Check in with yourself. How do you feel now?

Try it out when you first arrive at work or whenever you think you might be in for a stressful time during the day.

CHAPTER FIVE

STRESS TO CALM WITH HAPPINESS

Tip: Remember it's just ONE minute –
and you can CHOOSE happiness!

What's the lowdown?

The concept of choosing happiness involves recognising happiness as a choice that we can make in any moment, regardless of external circumstances. By changing our thoughts and focusing on positive emotions, we can move from feeling stressed to calm in a very short space of time. Posture can also play a role in this process, as adopting a more upright and confident posture can help to improve mood and reduce stress.

Studies have shown that choosing happiness and changing our state can have a range of benefits. One study published in *The Journal of Positive Psychology* found that simply recalling a positive memory for one minute can lead to significant increases in positive emotions and decreases in negative emotions. Another study published in the journal *Emotion* found that adopting a more upright and open body posture can increase feelings of power and confidence, leading to more positive emotions.

Engaging in positive activities, such as expressing gratitude or performing acts of kindness, can also lead to improvements in psychological wellbeing and reductions in stress.

By taking back control over our unconscious mind and changing our body posture to feel happier, we can improve our wellbeing and reduce stress in a short space of time.

> **'I am in charge of how I feel and today
> I am choosing happiness.'**
> Maya Angelou, civil rights activist and author

One very simple way of 'choosing happiness' is to consciously smile. This can be very powerful in reducing stress and improving your wellbeing.

In the film *Eat Pray Love*, taken from the book of the same name by Elizabeth Gilbert, you may remember the charming Medicine Man, who told Julia Roberts' character to smile. So smile! You can even try smiling – with your liver! We'll teach you how to do this in the Bonus Tool at the end of this chapter.

Smiling has a profound impact on our mental and physical health. Have you heard of the Facial Feedback Hypothesis? This suggests that the muscles involved in producing a smile can actually send signals to the brain, triggering the release of hormones and neurotransmitters associated with positive emotions. In other words, smiling can lead to the experience of happiness and wellbeing, even if it initially feels forced or inauthentic.

When we smile, our brain triggers a cascade of physiological responses that contribute to our overall wellbeing. Research has shown that the facial muscles involved in smiling send signals to the brain, stimulating the release of endorphins, dopamine and serotonin, which are the neurotransmitters associated with feelings of happiness, pleasure and relaxation. These natural 'feel-good' chemicals can counteract stress hormones such as cortisol, leading to a more tranquil state of mind.

Smiling not only influences our brain chemistry but also affects our body's stress response system. A study conducted by Kraft and Pressman (2012) revealed that even participants who were instructed to hold a 'forced' smile experienced a decrease in heart rate and a reduction in self-reported stress levels compared to a neutral facial expression. This suggests that the act of smiling can modulate our autonomic nervous system, promoting relaxation and calmness.

> **'Smile, breathe, and go slowly. Letting go gives us freedom, and freedom is the only condition for happiness.'**
> Thich Nhat Hanh

Amy Cuddy, a social psychologist and Harvard Business School professor, conducted a notable study on the power of smiling and its impact on stress reduction. In her research, Cuddy and her colleagues explored the concept of *fake it till you make it* by investigating whether the physical act of smiling, even if induced artificially, could influence an individual's stress response. The study involved participants holding a pencil between their teeth, to create a smile-like expression, while performing stressful tasks. The results of Cuddy's study were remarkable. Participants who maintained a forced smile, even with the pencil between their teeth, showed decreased stress levels compared to those who maintained a neutral facial expression. These findings suggest that the physical act of smiling, regardless of its authenticity, can have a genuine impact on reducing stress and promoting wellbeing.

Interestingly, the benefits of smiling extend beyond our individual experience. When we smile, we activate mirror neurons, which are specialised cells in our brain that mimic the facial expressions of others. These mirror neurons can trigger a positive feedback loop by prompting others to smile back, leading to a contagious effect of happiness and stress reduction. When we smile, and others smile back, we create a supportive environment.

So, the evidence is clear: smiling has the power to reduce stress and promote wellbeing. Even if it feels forced at first, the act of smiling can help create a positive feedback loop, leading to genuine feelings of happiness and wellbeing.

For this exercise we have combined smiling, breathing, a positive affirmation and a power pose so we get 4 for the price of 1 as it were!

TOOL 5

The Happy Exercise – give me just one minute!

Sitting or standing with good posture, close your eyes relax your arms by your side and take 5 relaxing breaths in and out.

Breathe in through your nose and exhale through your mouth. Remember to relax.

Do this 5 times, slowly and with intention.

Then to energise and to bring more happiness, confidence and success – *SMILE!* Smile big. Smile wide!

Open your eyes, place your hands in a fist by your shoulders or wherever is comfortable and then punch your arms upwards high in the air 10 times saying the positive affirmation **'well done'**. (You can say this silently or out loud.)

Well done, well done, well done, well done, well done!

(Keep smiling as you punch the arms in the air.)

Well done, well done, well done, well done, well done!

Repeat this exercise anytime you are stressed, at work, at home or even when you're out and about. OK, so you might get some looks if the hospital or surgery is busy, or you start punching the air walking down the corridor or at the bus stop, but as always … adapt to suit! Remember that just visualising you are punching the air is effective too!

At regular intervals during the day, when you become conscious of it, break into a smile, however daft it feels. Remember studies really have proven the power of the physiology of a smile.

Bonus Tool

If you want to choose to smile with different parts of your body – such as your liver – try this.

Breathe in and out and take notice of your flow of breath as you pay attention in your mind to your liver, near the bottom of your ribcage to the right, or to whichever part of your body you are imagining. Then notice how you feel as you imagine it smiling.

CHAPTER SIX

STRESS TO CALM AND THE POWER OF JOURNALING

Tip: Remember it's just ONE minute – and it's ONLY read by you!

What's the lowdown?

The act of writing down our thoughts, feelings and aspirations has been shown to have numerous benefits for our mental, emotional and even physical wellbeing in recent years. It's a simple yet profound practice that can allow us to let our thoughts flow and potentially unearth some thoughts and emotions that would otherwise remain hidden.

Journaling is the act of expressing our innermost thoughts and emotions through the written word. It provides a safe and private space for us to explore our desires, fears and dreams – without judgment or interruption. By putting pen to paper, we create a tangible reflection of our inner landscape, allowing us to gain clarity, discover patterns and unearth hidden treasures within ourselves. Notice we said, 'pen to paper', because it's definitely advantageous to write the old-fashioned way, by hand, rather than using a keyboard, because it's better for the cognitive brain.

Julia Cameron, a highly acclaimed author and creativity expert, has inspired millions of people to tap into their creative potential through her international bestselling book *The Artist's Way*. She introduces the practice of Morning Pages, a form of journaling where we are encouraged to write three pages of stream-of-consciousness thoughts each morning. Doing this daily makes it almost like a ritual, or a form of meditation, and it helps us to clear our mind, release self-doubt and negative talk onto the page (better out than in!) and even start to feel creative.

> **'Doing something that is productive is a great way to alleviate emotional stress. Gets your mind doing something that is productive.'**
> Ziggy Marley, musician

Writing our thoughts down without judgement, or editing, can help to alleviate stress and foster self-empowerment through positive affirmations. When we write about our worries, anxieties and frustrations, we externalise them, giving them less power over us. The mere act of acknowledging and articulating our stressors can bring a sense of relief and create space for problem-solving.

As Louise Hay, founder of Hay House Publishing, said, 'You can't clean the house till you can see the dirt.' If we are keeping it all hidden, it will be harder to deal with.

Journaling allows us to counteract negative self-talk by replacing it with positive affirmations. By intentionally affirming our worth, strengths and aspirations, we can cultivate a mind-set of self-compassion and resilience.

There is scientific evidence on the impact of journaling on wellbeing. A study conducted by Dr James W. Pennebaker, a leading researcher in the field of expressive writing, provides compelling evidence for the benefits of journaling. In his research, Dr Pennebaker found that individuals who engaged in expressive writing about their deepest emotions experienced significant improvements in their overall wellbeing. This included reductions in stress, improved immune function and enhanced psychological resilience. The study's findings highlight the transformative power of journaling as a therapeutic tool for personal growth and emotional healing.

So, grab a pen and a blank page and embark on the remarkable adventure of journaling. Your inner world and your inner power await!

TOOL 6

Grab a Pen and Journal – give me just one minute!

Here is a simple way of journaling while you are at home or at work, or even on the train, for one minute with positive affirmations.

1. Get a notebook or piece of paper – or maybe treat yourself to a special journal.//
2. Pick a positive affirmation and write it down – there's a list on the next page to help you get started.
3. Write about what the message means to you. Don't think too hard about this; write whatever comes into your mind straight away.

Keep an eye on the time so you spend only one minute – set a timer if needed.

You may find you jot down some rather random things, which is fine. You may come up with action steps or ideas, or it may encourage you to explore other things.

Write freely. Think about your body and your posture when writing and try to sit with good posture. You could even try the SMILE too!

Positive affirmations to choose from – or you can use one of your own.

I am loved, I am surrounded by love.

When negativity appears, I find a solution, talk to those I trust and think positively.

I love to smile; smiling makes me happy.

I am creative.

I am energetic.

I am healthy.

I have good relationships.

It's OK to be me.

I love setting goals.

I am peaceful.

I take breaks and rest to recharge my batteries.

I sleep well.

I am patient.

I breathe and relax.

I am calm.

I am enthusiastic.

I am OK with asking for help.

I am solution focused.

A Bonus Tool

You can extend this exercise by closing your eyes and visualising your goals or action steps that you are going to take; daydream about it. Afterwards, write down what came to you.

This exercise is another form of meditation and can be helpful in guiding you with decision making and planning in work and life in general.

If you enjoy journaling and would like to spend longer on this exercise, go for it! You could find this becomes a wonderful new regular practice.

CHAPTER SEVEN

STRESS TO CALM WITH SETTING GOALS AND VISUALISATION

Tip: Remember it's just ONE minute – and you can ACHIEVE your goals!

What's the lowdown?

Setting goals can be incredibly beneficial for both our work and personal lives. It gives us something to strive towards and helps us to focus our energy and efforts. Goals also give us a sense of purpose and motivation, and they can provide a framework for making decisions and prioritising tasks. We can't tell you what goals to set, but we can help you achieve them.

Research has shown that setting goals can be a powerful tool for personal and professional development. A study published in the *Journal of Applied Psychology* found that individuals who set specific, challenging goals performed better than those who set vague or easy goals.

Additionally, the study found that setting goals was associated with higher levels of motivation and job satisfaction (Locke and Latham, 2002).

> **'I am stronger than my challenges, and my challenges are making me stronger.'**
> Karen Salmansohn, behavioural change expert

Visualising the achievement of our goals can also have a powerful impact. This technique has been used by athletes and performers for decades to help them achieve their goals. By visualising ourselves successfully achieving our goals, we can create a mental blueprint that helps us to stay focused and motivated.

In the workplace most of us are aware of the **SMART** model to set effective goals: **S**pecific, **M**easurable, **A**chievable, **R**elevant and **T**ime-bound. Let's work with this model.

We need to start by thinking about what we want to achieve, our goal. Then break it down into smaller, manageable steps. Write it down, make it measurable within these steps, ensure it is achievable and realistic, and that it is relevant to what you want to achieve. Then put together a schedule of time in which you hope to achieve your goals. It's important to review this regularly to ensure you stay on track.

You may think this all sounds a bit 'corporate', if you are just trying to minimise stress and get through the day, but you can set goals for how you want to feel or respond to others or what you want in your personal life too. Some people worry that if they don't really have 'goals' or know what their 'purpose' is, they feel somehow that their life may not be meaningful. Far from it, as leading Hay House author and spiritual expert Kyle Gray says: *'Perhaps your purpose is just to be happy.'*

Imagine how that would ripple out if more people were content with themselves and their lives for being happy!

'You may not control all the events that happen to you, but you can decide not to be reduced by them.'
Maya Angelou

Incorporating visualisation into the goal-setting process is a way of focusing on how it will feel when you have accomplished what you have set out to do, and it is a great way of keeping motivated and focused.

We know that setting goals works, but when we incorporate visualisation it's especially powerful.

Feeling positive when we visualise our goals is important too. If we engage with positive self-affirmations, it can lead us to more optimism, greater happiness in our challenges and see less anger and less stress in the whole process.

TOOL 7

Reaching Your Goals and Seeing the Success – give me just ONE minute!

Sitting or lying down, close your eyes. You can even do this at a desk or on the train. Close your eyes and breathe and relax, breathing into your nose and out through your mouth.

Give yourself permission to think of a goal. This can be small or big – the ultimate big goal or part of the smaller steps to help achieve this. Choose something that is personal for you. It may just be a feeling you want to create more of.

Breathe in and out slowly and relax both your body and your mind.

Give yourself permission to see your goal, to hear what it sounds like, to feel it, to know something about it. Then breathe and relax, saying to yourself silently, *thank you for [this goal],* being explicit about what your goal is. Say thank you as if the goal has already been achieved. Enjoy this feeling of reaching your goal, this feeling of success.

Take a minute to do this and then open your eyes. Write down your chosen goal for this exercise and any insights that came to you during this time of visualising your goal and its success. These insights can be useful in helping you put small steps in place to make your visualisation a reality.

Are there any action steps that you need to take now to help you reach your goal?

CONCLUSION

CALM …

We really hope that you have enjoyed this book and have made the decision to try some or all the tools in your everyday life. We hope you are feeling calm.

> **'Calmness is the cradle of power.'**
> Josiah Gilbert Holland, author

Remember that reducing stress and anxiety in our lives is paramount to achieving good health and a fulfilling life.

Remember that reducing long-term stress can have a positive effect on our physical, mental and emotional health, and help us to prevent chronic illness and other health issues.

By incorporating simple stress-reducing tools into our daily routines, we can significantly improve our wellbeing and overall sense of calm and balance.

From breathing techniques, mindfulness practices, positive affirmations, stretching and goal setting, we have explored simple tools that can be easily incorporated into even the busiest of schedules. No excuses, not even for busy nurses!

These tools have been shown to have proven scientific benefits in reducing stress and anxiety, leading to improved overall health and happiness.

It is crucial to remind ourselves that taking care of our mental and emotional health is just as important as taking care of our physical health. By prioritising stress-reducing activities, we can lead a more balanced and fulfilling life, both at work and at home.

Remember, it's not what we do as a one-off that makes the difference; it's what becomes our daily 'self-care' practice. We urge you to implement these simple tools consistently and to achieve a healthier and happier life.

Remember, taking care of ourselves is a lifelong journey, and we owe it to ourselves to make our wellbeing a top priority. Selfcare is *not* selfish, it's 'showing up' to be the best you can be.

Remember to say: **Just give me ONE minute!** That one minute of time can make all the difference to your day.

We welcome feedback as to how these tools have worked for you, so please don't hesitate to get in contact. We are here for you.

Beverley and Janey

Here are some tips that help us when we are stressed.

Tips from Beverley

I love films, especially Christmas films! A relaxing way to switch off is to take outings to the cinema with my son.

To me, beach huts are paradise, there's nothing better than gazing out of a beach hut with the sight and sounds of the sea, having a picnic and swimming in the sea.

Resting and reading a good novel is a great form of escapism.

Pilates classes are fun and relaxing too.

Tips from Janey

I like taking myself off to an art gallery or an exhibition alone, no need to discuss how I feel about the art, I can just allow it to 'soak in' before hitting the café for coffee and cake.

If I'm feeling anxious, I've learnt to put in the PAUSE, breathe, and ask myself – in this moment am I ok? If the answer is yes, I'm safe and ok, if not, then I try and release the stress and do something soothing.

One of the best de-stressors is to put on a track you loved as a teenager and dance like no-one is watching … (hopefully they aren't!)

Tips for de-stressing from some of the nurses who responded to our survey.

I listen to podcasts to relax.

I try breathing exercises if I get stressed.

I decided to give up drinking alcohol.

Taking a five-minute break when feeling overwhelmed and going for a short walk. I find colouring in relaxing.

Being able to talk things through and vent frustrations helps me. Also doing a small burst of cardio exercise, i.e. a fast run on the spot raising knees high and pumping arms. I only need 30 seconds (a bit like a child throwing a paddy) but I feel so much better afterwards. By the time

Conclusion: CALM ...

my heart rate has settled down again I feel calmer and more relaxed. Not for in the middle of the ward obviously but try it on a trip to the toilet or canteen for lunch, or with a group of colleagues together outside – it usually causes a laugh within a group of you which also helps!

5 minutes stomping outside in fresh air for a small break at work helps. Yoga on my day off is always a winner.

And finally, why not write down some tips of your own!

ABOUT THE AUTHORS

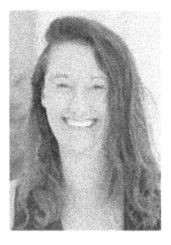

Beverley Densham, author of a number of books to include ***I Talk to Angels***, is an inspirational speaker and Mindfulness Pilates teacher and runs workshops and classes with her company Mindfulness Pilates. She works within law practices to promote the health and wellbeing of employees/lawyers. She regularly contributes articles to holistic and lifestyle magazines. She has a degree in Sports Science from University of Brighton.

www.beverleydensham.com

Linkedin @Beverley-densham

Instagram Beverley_densham

Twitter @BeverleyDensham

YouTube @mindfulnesspilates6603

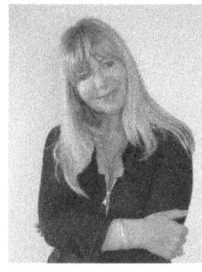**Janey Lee Grace** is an author and speaker. A former co-presenter on BBC Radio 2's *Steve Wright in the Afternoon* for 24 years, she was also a backing singer with Wham!, Kim Wilde and Boy George and had her own Number 8 chart hit as Cola Boy with '7 Ways to Love'. Janey has now written five books on holistic living, including the Number 1 Amazon bestseller ***Imperfectly Natural Woman***. Her latest book is ***Happy Healthy Sober***, which encourages everyone to look again at their relationship with alcohol.

www.janeyleegrace.com   www.thesoberclub.com

Linkedin @janeyleegrace

Instagram @janeyleegrace

Twitter @janeyleegrace

REFERENCES AND FURTHER READING

Introduction

Ghawadra, S.J. , Abdullah, K.J., Wan, Y.C., Mahmoud, D. and Cheng, K.P. 'The effect of mindfulness-based training on stress, anxiety, depression and job satisfaction among ward nurses: a randomized control trial', *Journal of Nursing Management*, 28(5) (2020) pp. 1088–1097.

1. Stress to Calm with Meditation

Creswell, J. D., Pacilio, L. E., Lindsay, E. K., and Brown, K. W., 'Brief mindfulness meditation training alters psychological and neuroendocrine responses to social evaluative stress', P*sychoneuroendocrinology*, 44, (2014), pp 1–12.

Epel, E. S., *et al,* 'Meditation and cortisol responses to stress: A randomized controlled trial', *Psychoneuroendocrinology* 68, (2016), pp 110–117.

Jerath, R., Edry, J. W., Barnes, V. A., and Jerath, V., 'Physiology of long pranayamic breathing: neural respiratory elements may provide a mechanism that explains how slow deep breathing shifts the autonomic nervous system', *Medical Hypotheses*, 67(3), (2006), pp 566–571.

Khoury, B., Sharma, M., Rush, S. E., and Fournier, C., 'Mindfulness-based stress reduction for healthy individuals: A meta-analysis', Journal of Psychosomatic Research, 78(6), (2015), pp 519–528.

Winfrey, O., 'The transformative power of meditation.' Oprah.com, (2013).

2. Stress to Calm with Positive Affirmations

Cascio, C. N. *et al.*, 'Self-affirmation activates brain systems associated with self-related processing and reward and is reinforced by future orientation', *Social Cognitive and Affective Neuroscience*, 11(4), (2016), pp 621–629.

Latham, G. P., and Locke, E. A., 'New Developments in and Directions for Goal-Setting Research', *European Psychologist*, 12(4), (2007), pp 290–300. https://doi.org/10.1027/1016-9040.12.4.290

Moser, J. S., Huppert, J. D., Duval, E., and Simons, R. F., 'Self-affirmation reduces cardiovascular reactivity to acute stress: Evidence from a real-world manipulation', *Journal of Health Psychology*, 35(9), (2016), pp 935–943

3. Stress to Calm with Neck and Shoulder Stretches

Jerath, R., Edry, J. W., Barnes, V. A., and Jerath, V., 'Physiology of long pranayamic breathing: neural respiratory elements may provide a mechanism that explains how slow deep breathing shifts the autonomic nervous system', *Medical Hypotheses*, 67(3), (2006), pp 566–571.

Pal, G. K., Velkumary, S., and Madanmohan, 'Effect of short-term practice of breathing exercises on autonomic functions in normal human volunteers', *Indian Journal of Medical Research*, 120(2), (2004), pp 115–121.

Telles, S., Singh, N., and Balkrishna, A., 'Heart rate variability changes during high frequency yoga breathing and breath awareness', *BioPsychoSocial Medicine*, 6(1), (2012), pp 1–7.

Zaccaro, A., *et al.*, 'How Breath-Control Can Change Your Life: A Systematic Review on Psycho-Physiological Correlates of Slow Breathing', *Frontiers in Human Neuroscience*, 12, (2018), p 353.

Zeidan, F., Johnson, S. K., Diamond, B. J., David, Z., and Goolkasian, P., 'Mindfulness meditation improves cognition: evidence of brief mental training', *Consciousness and Cognition*, 19(2), (2010), pp 597–605.

4. Stress to Calm with the Power stretch

Cuddy, A. J. 'Your body language may shape who you are', TED Talk, (2012). Retrieved from: https://youtu.be/Ks-_Mh1QhMc

Fredrickson, B. L., 'The Role of Positive Emotions in Positive Psychology: The Broaden-and-Build Theory of Positive Emotions', *American Psychologist*, 56(3), (2001), pp 218–226.

Fredrickson, B. L., Cohn, M. A., Coffey, K. A., Pek, J., and Finkel, S. M., 'Open hearts build lives: Positive emotions, induced through loving-kindness meditation, build consequential personal resources', *Journal of Personality and Social Psychology*, 95(5), (2008), pp 1045–1062.

Kruis, A., Tscharaktschiew, N., and Blanchard, C., 'Body posture effects on self-evaluation: A self-validation approach', *Emotion*, 18(4), (2018), pp 635–641.

5. Stress to Calm with choosing to Feel Happy

Abel, E. M., and Kruger, M. L., 'Smile Intensity in Photographs Predicts Longevity', *Psychological Science*, 21(4), (2010), pp 542–544.

Keysers, C., and Gazzola, V., 'Expanding the mirror: vicarious activity for actions, emotions, and sensations', *Current Opinion in Neurobiology*, 19(6), (2009), pp 666–671.

Kraft, T. L., and Pressman, S. D.,'Grin and Bear It: The Influence of Manipulated Facial Expression on the Stress Response', *Psychological Science*, 23(11), (2012), pp 1372–1378.

Soussignan, R. (2002) 'Duchenne smile, emotional experience, and autonomic reactivity', *Emotion*, 2(1), (2002), pp 52–75

6. Stress to Calm and the Power of Journaling

Pennebaker, J.W., 'Expressive Writing in Psychological Science', *Perspectives on Psychological Science*, 13(2), (2018), pp 226–229.

7. Stress to Calm with Setting Goals and Visualisation

Locke, E. A., and Latham, G. P., 'Building a practically useful theory of goal setting and task motivation: A 35-year odyssey', *American Psychologist*, 57(9), (2002), pp 705–717.

THE STRESS TO CALM IN 7 MINUTES SERIES

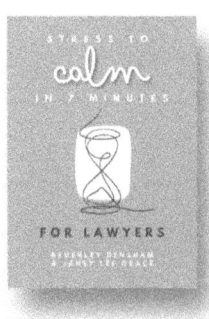 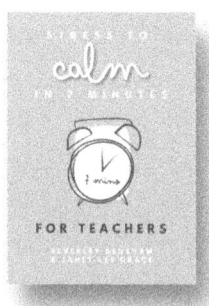 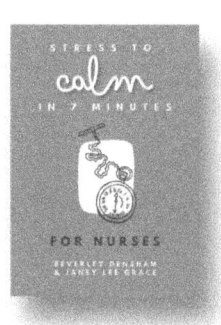

9780857162526 9780857162540 9780857162564

www.mcnidderandgrace.com

Milton Keynes UK
Ingram Content Group UK Ltd.
UKHW021154070124
435593UK00015B/90